The Gift of the Caregiver

The Gift of the Caregiver
by Julia Balzer Riley, RN, MN, HNC

Managing Editor
Susan Alvare

Editorial Assistant
Yvonne Gillam

Cover and Interior Design
Kirsten Browne

Page Layout
Kirsten Browne

H

Hartman Publishing
8529-A Indian School Road NE
Albuquerque, NM 87112
(505) 291-1274
www.**hartman**online.com

ISBN: 1-888343-65-6

PRINTED IN CHINA

THIS BOOK IS DEDICATED TO
A LIFE-LONG CAREGIVER,
BEVERLY DeMEO,
WHO WORKS HARD TO MAINTAIN
BALANCE IN HER LIFE WHILE
BRIGHTENING THE LIVES OF
OTHERS.

Days of darkness
Days of light.
Days of comfort
Days of fright.

Emotions felt
Beyond compare
The gift of life
A gift to care.

"My purpose in life is to be a caregiver," she told me. So many people review their lives and never feel connected to others, to life itself, but not this woman. For her mother, for her husband, for her community, she is a caregiver with love. She knows the gifts of the caregiver as do many women and men who choose to work at the bedside in long-term care, in home care, in hospitals and those who work behind the scenes to support caregiving. To be a caregiver is a gift. The caregiver receives many gifts along the winding journey. Caregivers are nursing assistants, home health aides, family caregivers, and others who provide safety, comfort and love to residents, clients and family members.

This book is a gift for caregivers with bits of wit and wisdom to nourish, inspire, and help you find the balance needed for the winding road of the journey. We, the author, the editor, the publisher, and all those whose stories and thoughts and experiences are shared here invite you to take a few minutes to read from this book in any order, whenever you want to be refreshed, to celebrate yourself and all the caregivers in your life. You enrich our lives, you save our lives, you bring joy and hope in times of despair and you laugh out loud at life's antics. We are truly grateful.

Within every problem there is a lesson. Release the problem and embrace the lesson.

Life is a series of problems to solve and it is from working through life's challenges that we grow. Next time a problem arises, instead of being put out by it, consider what life is trying to teach you.

I am in the right place at the right time doing the right thing in the right way.

"I braid her hair. She likes that." Wanda is a home health aide in Georgia who smiles with pride as she talks about a client she visited for a very long time. "We are like family."

What I can laugh at,
I can cope with.

Does your life ever seem out of your hands? Someone said having control of your life is like a toddler in the back seat, sitting in a car seat with a steering wheel, thinking he is driving the car. Give yourself the gift of a humorous perspective.

Laughter lightens the load.

Tom worked the evening shift and had a distinctive, joyful, full-body laugh. You would recognize it anywhere. When he laughed, we all laughed. We teased him endlessly about that laugh, but loved it. We needed his laughter. Share yours.

Plan something to anticipate with joy.

Fran, a friend who was also a nurse, loved pigs. I saw a magazine pattern for a pig pillow made of pink satin and decided to make it for her as a surprise. I had to enlarge a pattern, shop for the satin, and find pearls for eyes. Not having much time at night after work, it took a number of days to finish the project. But I anticipated my sewing time with joy, and it renewed my energy. What can you plan to anticipate with joy?

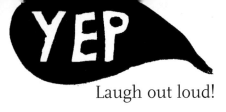

Laugh out loud!

How long has it been since you laughed out loud? What makes you laugh? Is it reruns of the *Three Stooges*? Do you have a favorite old movie? Do you have a favorite comedian? Do you laugh at humorous greeting cards? Add humor to your life so you can have a good laugh. Suggest that residents and clients select humorous videotapes or television shows. Laughter does a body good.

Humor helps.

A nursing assistant broke his leg and was forced to wear a cast. He got tired of answering the question, how did it happen? He had slipped on some water in his kitchen and was embarrassed. Finally when someone asked the question one time too many, he answered, "My boss appreciates my work so much that she throws rose petals at the door when I am coming in and I slipped and fell." A good laugh was had by all.

Laugh at yourself before somebody else does.

Have you ever tripped over you own feet and then looked around to see who was watching and would think you were clumsy? Next time, get up and laugh at yourself. People will think you have great poise and high self-esteem.

God has a sense of humor and I am giving Him some great material.

Next time you have a series of things that go wrong in your day, repeat this one liner to yourself. Humor helps us reframe how we see life and gives us back a sense of control.

Enjoy your inner giggle.

When you have to stand in lines, be a people watcher. Chuckle to yourself over a child at play. Look for things to make you smile. This is good practice in building your ability to find humor in life, which is an important skill for a caregiver.

Develop your comic vision.

A nurse manager keeps a pair of those big clown sunglasses in her desk. When the day is stressful for staff, she puts them on and walks down the hall. Everyone has a good laugh, takes a deep breath, and starts over.

Never let them see you sweat—think of how the Queen would handle it, or even Miss Manners.

In the middle of a divorce, one woman decided to keep her anger and sadness between her, her counselor, and a trusted friend. She had seen how a co-worker's resentment at an ex-spouse had damaged her reputation and made others around her uncomfortable. When she was tempted to say ugly things, she would ask herself how the Queen would conduct herself, chuckle, and move on. She slowly rebuilt her self-esteem by building new systems of support and she did not have to deal with embarrassment of past behavior.

> "I am free, I am unlimited.
> There are no chains to
> bind me."
>
> —FROM A HYMN

Find a song to sing. When things are tough, strengthen yourself with soothing, inspiring lyrics and melody. Hum quietly or sing to yourself in an empty hall at work. Let the song flow through your mind when you feel sad but still must get your work done. Ask residents and clients about their favorite songs and sing along.

An affirmation to repeat:
Centered and poised, I move
through this day easily and
gracefully.

Find a positive phrase of your own or use this one to overcome moments of fear or lack of confidence in yourself.

If you choose to eat dessert, slow down and savor each bite.

Sometimes we allow our guilt over a pleasurable treat to defeat the purpose. Make the good times last by paying attention.

Ask for a hug when you need one.
Offer a hug when it seems someone else needs one.

How we long for comfort and seem to forget that grown-ups need touch, too. Some people like hugs, others are more private. Just ask.

Only pick the weeds you can see from the road.

During a divorce, one woman found herself with less energy than usual. All the chores inside and outside the house fell to her now. Much of her energy was tied up in just getting to work and taking care of the children. So she learned sometimes to do just what has to be done right now!

Swinging on the refrigerator door is not an aerobic activity.

In Sue's family, they ate when they were happy, sad, angry or bored. Old bad habits are hard to break and in times of stress we may look for comfort in unhealthy behaviors or relationships— pay attention!

Schedule time for yourself.

As a caregiver, it seems as if everyone else's needs come first. You deserve a place on your own calendar. Plan to go to a movie, read a chapter in a novel, or take a long bath—whatever helps restore your energy.

It takes three trips to Ace Hardware.

Have you ever been trying to fix something and been frustrated when it didn't go smoothly? Rather than raging, try this philosophy. Next time you start a project and are on the way to the hardware store, tell yourself, "It takes three trips and this is number one."

When all else fails,
take a nap.

Judy's only relief in caring for her mother was
when the home health aide visited. She treated
herself to a brief nap. Sometimes it feels like our
brain is on overload. Even a 15-minute nap can
refresh you. Try taking a quick nap when you get
home from work.

When you are tired, take a nap.
Don't fight fatigue with food.

For those of us who use food for comfort, we may think a snack or a cup of coffee will be a pickup. Consider a brief walk at break time or getting to bed earlier. It is especially hard on the night shift when food seems to be everywhere. Pack your own dinner and healthy snacks so that cake isn't so tempting. When it is possible at home, take a nap.

M&M's call my name from the cupboard.

Yes! Sometimes chocolate *is* the answer.

Love your body as it is;
it serves you well.

We are so critical of our bodies. Too thin, too big, too tall, too short. Most people have some complaint about their bodies. A hospital volunteer had her picture taken for an identification badge. She thought her face looked too round. The photographer commented, "You look so healthy." This made the woman stop and think.

So many of our clients can no longer do the things we take for granted. Take a moment to be grateful for your health. Celebrate yourself just as you are. When you learn to love your body, you naturally take better care of it.

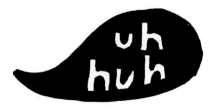

uh
huh

I don't have to buy everything I like. It usually requires dusting.

Life as a caregiver is stressful. Ever get mall fever—when everything is something you "can't live without"? Well, you can! Be a window shopper and a people watcher instead. At bill time you will thank yourself.

I can't always control what happens to me, but I can control my response to it.

Sometimes life seems unfair and out of control, herein lies your power. Victor Frankl, a prisoner of war, said, "They can do that they will to my body, but they can't affect my mind." Each day he looked for a chance to do something good for someone else and in his mind he wrote his famous book, *Man's Search for Meaning*.

Are you your own worst critic? Lighten up!

If self-esteem is how you see yourself compared to how you would like to be, one way to raise your self-esteem is to lower your standards.

I know God sends us this stuff so we can grow, but haven't I grown enough for a while?

It is okay to just be down and overwhelmed sometimes. Feelings are neither good or bad; they just are! Take that nap.

No matter where you live, it is a small town. Speak ill of no one, because you never know who is sitting in the booth behind you.

A home health aide went out to dinner at a restaurant with good home cooking and large booths. She was with a close friend visiting from out of town. The aide was describing her tough day with a difficult client to her friend. As they walked out to pay, she saw the client's mother was in the next booth—a woman she admired. Fortunately, she had not used the client's name, although she had given specific details. She didn't know if the mother had heard or if she knew that her son was the client being discussed. The aide felt her face get red and quickly left the restaurant, having learned a valuable lesson.

Watch what you say and where you say it.

Never say anything bad about the company that employees you. That is who writes your paycheck, and, the boss might be in that booth behind you in the restaurant! Work within the company to change it. Don't take your complaints outside. This is called loyalty.

Before you repeat it, ask yourself if you would say it if the person was in the room.

Ouch! Gossip is so tempting! Resist that temptation. They could be talking about you next week. Just take the high road and just say no to tacky tales.

When life gets tough, wear purple underwear.

No one needs to know. You will feel great and have a smile on your face all day.

Ask for what you want. Don't expect that "if he loves me, he will know what I want."

If a man buys a woman a black nightie and it is too small, he's in BIG trouble. If a man buys a woman a black nightie and it is too big, he is in BIG trouble. Be specific or go shopping with him.

Just say "NO" to cynicism.

Are you tired of negative people spoiling your coffee break? Try this next time: "I'm trying hard to stay positive and it is hard, isn't it? Would you like me to tell you what helps me?"

If you don't know you are wonderful, who else will?

Sandra was always saying negative things about herself. It made other staff uncomfortable. Avoid putting yourself down. It is unattractive and a real turn-off. Instead, treat yourself well and expect others to also. You are one-of-a-kind.

"I may not be totally perfect, but parts of me are excellent."

—Ashley Brilliant

Okay, so I'm not perfect and you're not perfect either. Yes, I take responsibility for my mistakes, but I can lighten up a bit. I don't have to be paralyzed from my mistakes. I can learn from them to improve my work. And I will remember to notify my boss of any mistakes, rather than letting him or her hear it from someone else.

Courage is fear that has said its prayers.

Her father's progressive memory loss and deterioration was so painful. He had been a proud military officer and now couldn't remember to bathe. She found that expressing herself in poems helped. Sometimes she wrote prayers. Caregivers need time for reflection and for remembering.

Nature heals.

Betty always felt closest to a Higher Power when she was outside. She made it a point to go outside for a break. She would sit alone quietly and say a prayer of gratitude for her own life and the privilege of serving others. The power of nature humbled her and added perspective. How can you add time with nature to your day?

Each of us has a limited amount of mental energy— worry wisely!

Ann worked in long-term care and comforted residents and family with a favorite one-liner. "I'm your designated worrier so you can RELAX. I'm worrying enough for you and me both!" Then they could talk about how seldom things we worry about come true. Take life one moment at a time.

If you are sick, be sick.

If you have a cold or the flu, do us all a favor and stay home and take care of yourself. Rest, eat your comfort foods, and take it easy. You deserve it and we don't want to be sick either!

Feel the fear and do it anyway.

—SUSAN JEFFERS

If we wait until we aren't afraid to try something new, we just won't grow. Susan Jeffers recommends taking those little yellow sticky notes, writing "I can handle it" on them, and putting them all over the house.

F.E.A.R. is Forgetting Everything is All Right.

—JACQUELYN ALDANA

Most of those things we worry about never happen anyway. Use this phrase to remind yourself.

Just do it!

Consider this well-known slogan for shoes. Start things one step at a time. Put one foot in front of the other. That's how we get stuff done.

Dress up! You will feel better.

Pay attention to your grooming. Wear the clothes that make you feel your most attractive, yet professional. People notice if your clothes are clean and pressed, and this makes a statement about how you value yourself. One nurse's sixth grade son complained to his mother that the teacher seemed to be picking on him. The mother had allowed him to wear baggy shirts with skateboarding emblems. She suggested they try an experiment. For several days, he wore clean short-sleeved shirts with collars and reported that things went more smoothly at school. Whose behavior was affected? The teacher's from a different impression? The child's from feeling more grown-up? Or both?

"I think I can. I think I can. I think I can."

—FROM *THE LITTLE ENGINE THAT COULD*

Tina used to read her children this story. One day at work she caught herself thinking discouraging thoughts. She laughed out loud as she caught herself. She thought of that bedtime story she had read her daughter the night before. She decided if it's good enough for that little train, it's good enough for her.

Any resentment you hold towards another will do that person very little harm but will destroy you.

John had not gotten the promotion he thought he deserved and found himself angry with his coworker who had gotten the job. He brooded about it. It corrupted his day and drained his energy. Why do we think not forgiving someone or being upset with him "serves them right" when it actually serves us so badly?

Not forgiving someone is like stabbing yourself in the stomach to hurt the person standing behind you or drinking poison to poison someone else.

Get the picture?

Let go and let God. He does a better job anyway.

One day when I was having trouble forgiving a troublesome person in my life, my aunt told me a story about an old woman who packed all her troubles into a battered suitcase and carried them up the mountain to God. She asked Him to take her burdens. He agreed to do so, but she just couldn't help herself. She picked up that heavy suitcase and dragged it back down the mountain. I realized I had been allowing my energy to be drained by a person and just needed to let go.

To deal with a lack of forgiveness, wish for happiness and prosperity and health for the other; all the wonderful things you would wish for yourself.

What a light feeling. How good you feel—almost smug for being so good. What a big person you are. This is good for the soul and it works.

Forgive, but don't forget.

Sometimes we find ourselves being taken advantage of by someone we know. For our own good, we learn the lesson and forgive ourselves and the other person. However, next time this person tries to get us to do something that is not in our best interests, we remember and nicely, but firmly, refuse to be taken in again.

Bitterness is tacky and unattractive.

I knew a woman who moved me to tears when she talked about the pain of her divorce. Such sympathy I felt until I found out her divorce was 17 years ago. She was still angry at this man, frequently angry at work, and spoke harshly to others. My mother used to say, "Don't make an ugly face; it might freeze that way." I thought of this whenever I worked with this woman. It seemed she had a permanent frown on her face. Her bitterness caused other people to avoid her. If you find you can't let go of anger, find a counselor, someone at employee health, or a member of the clergy to work through this. Unresolved anger is bad for your health.

If you have a partner, go home and make love. There are so many people who are alone who have no one with whom to be intimate.

Of course, sexuality is a complicated issue for many people. Yet, sometimes that isn't the problem. We just get busy and forget that both men and women have sexual needs and that making love can be a great comfort.

Touch your loved one often and lovingly.

Treasure your partner. Pay attention to touch.

Snuggle with your partner.

I am remarried and try not to take this precious man for granted. We use the snooze alarm on our clock radio. I put my head on his shoulder. It is such a peaceful feeling and a good way to start our day.

No one is irreplaceable. Take care of your body. One to a customer, you know.

If you die young from overwork, no one will name a bridge after you. They will kick your worn body aside, hire two young ones, and pay them more.

No man on his deathbed ever said, "I wish I had spent more time at work."

Our children are with us such a short time. Cherished loved ones die. Today make plans to spend time with someone who is important to you.

The loose valve theory: as we age those valves in our bodies that keep us from making tacky body noises loosen, and we can't help ourselves.

Learn to laugh at yourself and with others. We are all in this together.

When I can't remember what I was saying, just give me a clue and be patient, I am having a menopausal moment.

Be patient with people who are older than you. If you are lucky, you will get older too.

When I can't find my glasses, that is a senior moment.

This is not a sign of early senility. We are busy and get distracted.

Aging does not trouble me because I know I am chronologically gifted.

Change your words. Change your attitude.

"I went to bed one night with a waist, and woke up the next morning without one."

—A BELOVED MOTHER-IN-LAW

Our bodies change and humor helps.

I want wisdom
and I want it now.

Elders are a rich resource of life experience. Make
friends with people older than you. Encourage
residents/clients to share their stories.

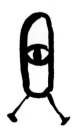

When you are angry or frustrated, take to the streets and walk or jog.
It is impossible to be angry and short of breath at the same time.

Don't be overcome by the power of anger. Harness that power in a healthy way.

In the face of anger consider this: anger is a response to frustration, a sense of powerlessness, and a fear of the loss of control.

This idea can change how you see anger. It can make you want to understand rather than lash out with your anger.

To have a friend, be a friend.

Invest in friendships. Call, write, email, or visit. Make yourself available to friends in a crisis. Make plans today to see a friend to have time to enjoy each other.

The best "conversationalist" is one who speaks little and listens earnestly.

How wonderful to find someone interested in what you think and feel—a sure sign of intelligence.

"God gave us two ears and one mouth for a reason."

—Mary Kay Ash

Cindy, a home health aide, offered the following advice to new aides. "Keep your sense of humor and listen to your patients' stories, especially older patients. They have a lot to teach us." Cindy's favorite one-liner is "It's what you learn after you know it all that counts."

If you don't like your relatives, adopt a few new ones or a few extras if your family is small.

As an only child, I longed for a brother or sister. A nurse friend took care of me when I had surgery, spending several nights at my house so my young son would not worry. She had always longed for a sister, too. As I write, I sip water from a mug she gave me which says, "Soul Sister #1—trusted accomplice, disaster counselor, and love advisor." She and her husband became my son's aunt and uncle and we have joined them for Thanksgiving dinner on many occasions; family is not just through genetics!

uh huh

And speaking of mugs—

Choose your coffee cup by your mood, to wallow in it or get over it. I have one that says "Snap out of it" and an Oscar the Grouch one for when I am not ready to get over my mood. Another says "Joy". Find the cup that suits you.

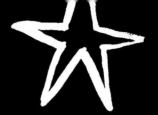

She was a legend in her own mind.

Say less about your accomplishments. Let others sing your praises.

He was a legend in my own mind.

Sometimes we endow people with the traits we wish they had. Have you ever been disappointed when people did not live up to your idea of them? Maybe you were wearing "rose-colored" glasses at the time. See people as they really are.

Beware of promises and apologies that follow violent behavior.

Love is a verb. We know behavior speaks louder than those promises of never-again. Every man, woman and child has the right to live without fear of physical, emotional, or sexual abuse.

If he seems to be too good to be true, he probably is.

If she seems to be too good to be true, she probably is.

Look for a RP—real person. Real people don't look perfect or act perfectly but they do grow on you in time. Use your head. Everyone has flaws. It is better to know which ones now than later.

Children most need love when they are the most unlovable.

I saw this on a poster of a parent comforting a furious child. "Will you still love me when I misbehave? Do I have to misbehave to get your attention?" Next time my little one pitched a fit, I asked him if he wanted me to leave or stay. He shouted, "stay!" I think that poster must have been right.

To reach the tender leaves,
the giraffe must stick his
neck out.

Have you thought about going back to school,
but were afraid you couldn't finish the program?
You'll never finish if you don't even start.

Learn to tolerate silences.
Someone else may have
something important to say.

Breathe. Some people talk to fill any silence
because silence makes them nervous. Silence can
be productive. Some people need time to think
before they speak.

The enemy of the good
is the better.

Jane had gone back to school and was faced with her first writing assignment. She feared she couldn't write an "A" paper. A friend told her a story of someone who failed her assignment because she never turned in a paper. Her friend reminded her that it was better to turn a paper in rather than have none for fear of lack of perfection. So Jane sat down and got started.

> "If you think you can, you can. And if you think you can't, you're right."

—MARY KAY ASH

Mr. D was not easy to care for. No one seemed able to please him. John, a CNA, said that he knew the resident was uncomfortable and scared. John got to work a few minutes early and started having his coffee with Mr. D. They swapped stories and jokes. Caregivers learn that sometimes you get what you expect from people.

> "Advice is what we ask for when we already know the answer but wish we didn't."

—ERICA JONG

Everyone needs a friend who will give an honest answer even if it's what you don't want to hear. That takes courage.

Resist the urge to shut down emotionally. Start over and take the risk to build intimacy in your life.

Joan wanted a close relationship with her dad but his demands on her were increasing. She lived close and did errands since he no longer drove. She knew if she did not set some limits she would grow to resent him. She had the courage to talk about her need to run all the errands on one day a week and he started making a list. Honest communication is a part of intimacy.

"The dedicated life is worth living. You must give with your whole heart."

—ANNE DILLARD

Mr. G likes his water without ice and Mrs. C likes her water full of ice. Tom takes pride in remembering his residents' preferences because he knows it gives them a sense of control. Tom is passionate about his work and his life. We need more enthusiasm around us. It's attractive and contagious and is a people magnet.

"It is not easy to find happiness in ourselves, and it is not possible to find it elsewhere."

—AGNES RIPPLIER

Ann's role as caregiver sometimes leaves her resentful. She has other brothers and sisters. Yet she is the one who has assumed the full-time role as caregiver for their mother. It is easy to blame them but she has found it doesn't help. She has learned to honor her decision. In accepting she is there by choice, she finds peace.

"Life is the first gift,
love is the second, and
understanding is the third."

—Marge Piercy

Appreciate your life, the people in your life, and
the lessons life provide.

Life is a miracle; embrace it.

Working with people who are sick or who are
dying is a wake-up call. Cherish each day. Each
one is numbered. What are you doing with today
that you would want to remember?

Life is full of wonder.
Are you looking for it?

Color in a flower blooming, the smell of bread baking, the sound of a bird singing, or the touch of a friend.

Is life a problem to solve or a mystery to unravel?

Maybe not knowing what will happen is a good thing. Expect a miracle.

"Tired? Remember, there will be plenty of time to rest in the home."

—SUE BALE

That's what a friend of mine said at the time of life where we were both managing toddlers. She's right. Plan now to stay up late to do something fun.

"If you don't know where you
are going, any path will do."

—FROM *ALICE IN WONDERLAND*

Research shows that people who write down their
goals are much more likely to achieve them.

Surround yourself with flowers. Smell one today.

Put beauty in your life on purpose. Buy a few flowers at the grocery store or put some wild flowers in a vase. If you have a garden, share flowers at work. Taking a moment to enjoy the beauty in nature relaxes, refreshes, and helps us have a positive attitude.

Life is too short to use cheap napkins.

We all have pet peeves or preferences. Cheap napkins are for pizza or picnics. Setting a pretty table is important to me and so I give myself permission to buy soft paper napkins or use cloth ones. What can you do where you work and live to fulfill your need for beauty?

Any dinner looks better by candlelight.

We can make everyday events a celebration. Don't wait for someone else to do it. Make life special.

Have a room or a corner or a shelf to display your treasures—a pretty found object, a picture from a child.

You don't have to have a lot of money to have beauty and order in your life and, if you find out how to have order, call me first.

Take a mental vacation.

The brain doesn't know the difference between
being in Hawaii and pretending to be there.
Take a few minutes to go somewhere beautiful in
your mind.

When there is a choice, take
the scenic route.

Nature is soothing. Take advantage of this natural
medicine. If you can't have a window at work, try
hanging a landscape painting. We did that for the
small space where our phone operators work. It
added calm in the midst of chaos.

Remember the Platinum Rule: "Do unto others as they would have you do unto them."

A couple married. In the husband's family when people were sick, they left each other alone for privacy. In the wife's family, people fussed over the sick and brought chicken soup. When the wife got sick, her husband practiced the golden rule and left her alone. She thought he didn't care about her. Let others know what you want. Don't assume everyone is like you.

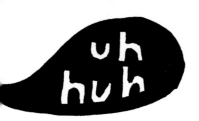

When in doubt, be still and listen.

When the child of a friend died, there were no words and none were necessary. Presence in the face of suffering is the greatest gift.

"Seek first to understand, then to be understood."

—STEPHEN COVEY

Your own point of view, which you were busy rehearsing, might change.

Communication is what is received, not what was intended.

If you are not sure the other person understood what you meant, ask the person to repeat what he heard you say.

Don't pout. It won't get you chocolate ice cream.

Sometimes when someone we work with hurts our feelings, we want to avoid them even when an apology is offered. If this happens, consider the story of a three-year-old child who wanted chocolate ice cream but her parents said "no." She stomped off and refused the ice cream when her mother later softened and offered it. Later she realized she had her pride, but no ice cream.

Speak your love.
Write your love.
Live your love.

Anne applied hot pink nail polish. When she had a few spare moments, Anne helped Mrs. S to get ready for her grandson's visit. They knew he always noticed any changes and worked together to surprise him. Caregivers develop a rich history with long-term clients and use it to make special connections.

Talk less.
Communicate more.

Terese cleaned the glass on the salad bar table near closing time in the hospital café. She called to a lone customer, "You're here every night, aren't you?" The woman talked softly about her son who was paralyzed from Guillian Barre's syndrome. All the staff in the hospital were caregivers.

Consistency builds trust.

Hospice was his lifeline. When his pain was out
of control or when he just didn't "feel right," he
placed a call and waited with quiet confidence.
"She'll call right back. She always does."
Caregivers can be depended upon and their
word is a sacred bond.

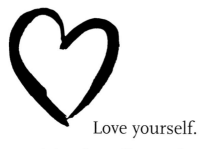

Love yourself.

As I care for myself, so I care for my patients.
As I care for myself, so I care for the families.
As I care for myself, so I care for my coworkers.

The antidote for talking a lot is measured words.

It has been said that we have 15,000 thoughts each day. There is no need to share each one.

Never hurry. Never worry.

After breakfast, Joann always took a moment to make sure everything her patient needed was close at hand. She remembered to ask, "Is there anything else you need before I go?" Caregivers anticipate a patient's needs.

Listen for the unspoken.

"They are so kind to me and always seem to know what I need." Mrs. H needed help at home after her stroke. The homemaker services and visits from the aides and nurses made it possible for her to remain at home surrounded by 50 years of family memories. A team of caregivers working together supported and inspired her and added years to her life. They trusted their intuition in ways to personalize her care.

"Marriage is ups and downs, but mostly plateaus."

—SUE BALE

Marriage is a commitment to live life together in good times and bad times and when the dishes are dirty. Our commitments may be challenged when the role of caregiver is added. We need to look to our history together to sustain us and learn that our love can take a new form and shape in daily hands-on caregiving.

Put your spouse and your children on your calendar.

We write in our calendar what is important. Review your calendar and see if what you value shows up anywhere on the pages. If not, take time right now, set aside some time for loved ones and negotiate some time with them.

Are you looking for answers? Be still and pray or meditate.

Today I will walk outside alone and pay attention to nature. I will thank God for all the things for which I am grateful. I will present my problem to God and ask for the solution that is for the greatest good of all involved.

"Nature, time, and patience are three great physicians."
—CHINESE PROVERB

Mike works as an aide in a long-term care facility. He takes time to fish each week and laughs when people ask him if he has caught anything. He knows that the fishing pole is an excuse to just sit and soak up the majesty of nature. It soothes his soul.

"And if not now, when?"
—THE *TALMUD*

Caroline is a caregiver in a hospice house and appreciates each day of her own life, speaking of her work as a blessing in her life. She makes it a point to see dear friends regularly because she knows tomorrow might not come.

> Today I will spend five minutes alone and in silence and begin to really listen.

Two strategies for success: Pray and Play.

Today I will remember to say a prayer for myself and for others in my life. I will plan something fun to do to renew my energy and help me have a fresh start.

Something wonderful is about to happen.

It takes courage to take a deep breath and tell
yourself, "Everything will work out."
We all need courage.

We are all connected.

Rita reminds herself that she could be the one whose speech has been slurred by a stroke and each day she pays attention to slowing her own speech and encouraging her patient to speak.

Consider your work a sacred path.

Susan always took an extra moment to make physical contact. Mrs. P remembered that touch on her arm and felt its warmth long after Susan left the room. Caregivers know that people feel lonely and for some, a gentle touch is a reminder that they are lovable.

We are all family.

Donna's grandchildren were the twinkle in her eye so she talked easily with patients about theirs and admired pictures at the bedside. She shared the latest knock-knock jokes with patients who groaned in delight at the corny humor. Caregivers know that humor helps.

There is no such thing as false hope.

Justine was often asked by her patients to pray with them. She would pray for peace and comfort. Today I will speak words of hope and look for the positive in every situation.

Just say "Thank you."

Have you noticed that if you pray, you are often asking for something? Stop for a moment, close your eyes, take a deep breath, and just say "thank you" for all you have. This can reframe your whole day.

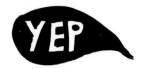

Someone always sees.
Someone always knows.

Janet, a CNA, worked steadily with a sense of
satisfaction through one of those never-ending
evening shifts, remembering the smile on one
patient's face when she had presented the patient
with her favorite caffeine-free diet soda. The
hospital stocked a different brand. Janet knew
that little things do mean a lot.

I am allowed high standards for myself.

Sometimes it seems like it isn't "cool" to do your best or say "no" to something that does not seem right. Remember we come into this world alone and leave the same way. "Cool" doesn't matter then.

You get what you expect. Raise your expectations.

Mary's role as a caregiver for her sister has become so time consuming that she sometimes feels she has forgotten who she is. She refuses to let that happen so she takes a moment to walk outside, take a deep breath, and say a prayer for the greatest good for all involved.

I am uncertain about the future, but I am certain it is positive.

Everyone who walked by the nurses' station seemed to take time to smell the fragrant bouquet of homegrown roses Tonya brought to work. Caregivers share their gifts and talents to brighten the day of coworkers.

Assume an attitude of gratitude.

Sandra seemed to be the family caregiver and was sometimes overwhelmed with the responsibility. In a support group she shared the idea of a gratitude journal that she kept faithfully. Whenever she got scared or sad she could read it and start over again.

Attitudes are the crayons with which we color our lives.

John, a long-time employee in housekeeping, buffed the hospital floors in the early morning hours. When asked about his work, he spoke with pride. "If people see these floors are clean, and well-cared for, they know we all take pride in our work." John was a part of the healthcare team and knew his contribution was valuable.

Attitudes are contagious. Is yours worth catching?

Be the person people look forward to seeing coming down the hall. Smile and greet people warmly. You don't have to like everybody. If you are shy, just smile.

You never know how you affect people.

Frank worked in our maintenance department and we joked with each other whenever we met. One day, I was having a very sad day. I had just presented a motivational program for staff—my job—even though I didn't feel like it. When I looked up, I saw Frank had been watching me and had stopped to hold the door. I asked him why. He said, "You just looked like you needed a good turn." I have never forgotten Frank and I tell the story over and over.

Take your work professionally, not personally.

You don't have to like everything you have to do, but no one else has to know that.

> "Coincidences are just God's way of working a miracle anonymously."

A favorite bumper sticker

When you expect a miracle, you might just get one.

Whine not, want not!

Just don't do it. No one likes to hear whining. When you complain over and over about the same things and refuse to do anything about them, you are not producing solutions. If you are unhappy with your life, change it, accept it, or find a professional counselor to work on it.

If the words, "I told you so" bubble up in your throat, stifle yourself!

Wait until you are asked for your opinion. Just because someone tells a story incorrectly or has the facts mixed up, doesn't mean you have to correct them unless it's life or death.

How much personality can I have if everyone likes everything I do?

It just is not possible to please everyone.
Be selective.

Be persistent.

Few people get something right the first time.
Keep trying and practice, practice, practice.

Be careful about what you put into your consciousness.

Remember the old computer saying: garbage in equals garbage out. Read uplifting stories. Watch a funny movie rather than a violent and gory one.

"Most people are about as happy as they make up their mind to be."

—ABRAHAM LINCOLN

Linda's mother had open-heart surgery and talked about wanting her "blues" to go away. She was distressed because she could not explain her sadness. Linda found a beautiful bubble blower and bought bubble solution. Together they blew bubbles and laughed. Her mother still uses that bubble blower when she wants to brighten her day.

Having married an Irishman, I would like to end
with an Irish blessing:

May the road rise up to meet
you.

May the wind always be at
your back.

May the sun shine warm
upon your face.

May the rain fall soft upon
your field.

And until we meet again,

May God hold you in the
hollow of His hand.

The Gift of the Caregiver is a product of over 25 years of facilitating caregivers' professional and personal growth—a legacy from a psychiatric nurse and professional speaker, Julia Balzer Riley, RN, MN, HNC, who believes, "If I can laugh at it, I can cope with it."

Contact Julia at Julia@ConstantSource.com or 1-800-368-7675. Visit her website at www.ConstantSource.com.